Lactation Management:

Strategies for Working with African-American Moms

By Katherine Barber
CLEC, Breastfeeding Advocate

Lactation Management:

Strategies for Working with African-American Moms

Katherine Barber, CLEC, Breastfeeding Advocate

Praeclarus Press, LLC

2504 Sweetgum Lane

Amarillo, Texas 79124 USA

806-367-9950

www.PraeclarusPress.com

DISCLAIMER

The information contained in this publication is advisory only and is not intended to replace sound clinical judgment or individualized patient care. The author disclaims all warranties, whether expressed or implied, including any warranty as the quality, accuracy, safety, or suitability of this information for any particular purpose.

ISBN: 9781939807915

Dedication/Acknowledgements

As always, each word has its root in the birth of my two angels here on earth. This and all words I am blessed to have published are dedicated to A and J.

My family, my friends, my advocates – I give thanks for your motivation and encouragement.

To my editor's patience, thanks *ad infinitum.*

To breastfeeding professionals everywhere, your work is invaluable.

Table of Contents

Introduction

Why am I qualified to write this book? I am an African-American mother who has successfully breastfed. I have a La Leche League background. Because of the lack of breastfeeding resources in the African-American community, I started the African American Breastfeeding Alliance (AABA). And, I've written a book – *The Black Woman's Guide to Breastfeeding*.

For well over ten years, I have had the pleasure of educating breastfeeding peer counselors, certified lactation counselors, certified lactation education counselors, La Leche League Leaders, registered nurses, medical doctors, and others on the nuances of breastfeeding in the African-American community.

With the birth of my first child in 1997, I began my personal journey into the world of breastfeeding. It was a journey I did not plan to embark on, other than to nurture my son in the best way possible. However, the universe had other plans. I nursed him for two years and became pregnant with my daughter, who I nursed for 17 months. While I had minimal breastfeeding problems and a family who encouraged me, I still sought out the company of other African-American women. Unfortunately, I could not find any Black support groups in or outside of my community. The only support I found were a few breastfeeding classes in the WIC program, which I was not enrolled in.

My first book, *The Black Woman's Guide to Breastfeeding: The Definitive Guide to Nursing for African American Mothers,* was birthed from my breastfeeding experiences. It was a culmination of many things. First, breastfeeding my children left an impression on me that compelled me to help other women in my community to breastfeed their own babies. Second, founding the African American Breastfeeding Alliance (AABA – a nonprofit organization designed to educate African-American families about the importance of breastfeeding) in January of 2000 and running it for over seven years helped to create a national groundswell among women, government, and private agencies about the urgent need to reach Black women with the breastfeeding message. Finally, the health of Black babies was and still is in a pandemic state. I had to do my small part to make a difference. My small part was to educate women about breastfeeding.

I am writing this book to help lactation and other professionals provide effective and culturally specific lactation services to African-American women. The one question that has been consistent in my work has come from lactation professionals of other races. They want to know, "How do I reach African-American women?"

This book is one tool for them to add to their resource library. It is my hope that this will not just help the reader reach Black women and provide better lactation services, but will ultimately make a difference in the health of Black mothers and babies.

Chapter One.
African-American Women and Breastfeeding - Statistics

The United States is arguably the most powerful country on the global scene – providing unsurpassed opportunities and freedom for its citizens, technology advancements, and influencing the economy of other nations. That said the U.S. still falls short when it comes to the health of its mothers and infants. In the area of lactation, we are on shakier ground and divided racially. Breastfeeding is not the cultural norm in the U.S. An even closer examination shows the cultural landscape of breastfeeding here is decidedly divided by race.

The American Academy of Pediatrics (AAP) recommends, "Exclusive breastfeeding for approximately the first six months and support for breastfeeding for the first year and beyond as long as mutually desired by mother and child" (AAP, 2012). However, according to the Centers for Disease Control (CDC), of the infants born in the U.S., 75% are breastfed at birth (CDC, 2012). The study does not conclude that the 75% breastfed were done so exclusively. In fact, among children born in 2007, 43% were breastfeeding at six months and 22% at 12 months of age – a major decrease from initiation. And of those who continued breastfeeding, a supplement of infant formula was a large part of the feeding process.

African-American women have the lowest breastfeeding rates in the United States. Only 59.7% of African-American women breastfeed according to the CDC study (CDC, 2012). It's important to note that this rate means that 59.7% of African-American women attempt to breastfeed – not that they breastfeed exclusively or for a specific period of time. By three, six, and 12 months, the rates drop off drastically, with 27.9% breastfeeding at six months and 12.9% still breastfeeding at 12 months (CDC, 2012). It is vital to promote breastfeeding to the African-American community and provide effective lactation counseling. The health of Black babies is at risk.

African-American infants are twice as likely to die before their first birthdays as white infants (MacDorman & Mathews, 2008). African-American infants/children have some of the highest rates of asthma, severe asthma, and mortality caused by asthma (National Heart Lung and Blood Institute, 2012). And they have a 20% higher occurrence of childhood obesity than white children (DHHS, 2012a). These are just a few of the health gaps that exist in the African-American community that can be greatly reduced, or almost eradicated, if breastfeeding rates are increased; not to mention the reduction in health factors for African-American women, namely premenopausal breast cancer (American Cancer Society, 2012; DHHS, 2012b).

Guiding Principle: Recognize the cultural landscape of breastfeeding and the barriers African-American women experience as an important element in lactation management.

Chapter Two.
History of Breastfeeding and African-American Women

When seeking to understand the totality of a Black woman's breastfeeding choices and experiences, it's key to look at her history. African-Americans were once the premier breastfeeding population here and in Africa. We did not always have the lowest breastfeeding rates. In fact, breastfeeding is deeply rooted in African history. What was once a normal, natural part of mothering for African women radically changed when they were brought to America as slaves. Slavery dramatically changed the course of mothering and breastfeeding for African-American women. (Note: The history will focus largely on the areas of West Africa where most African Americans originate).

> Whenever I speak publicly about breastfeeding and African-American women, I always bring to light a historical perspective. You have to know where you've been to know where you're going. This adage has been said from the Ancient Chinese philosophers to African sayings, even to Winston Churchill.

Before coming to this country as slaves (more than 250 years ago), African women had 100% breastfeeding rates – exclusive breastfeeding from birth provided optimal child spacing. There is no evidence of breastmilk substitutes on the African continent pre-slavery to date. However, due to slavery and its resulting division of the Black family, wet nursing, the Great Migration, and infant formula, African-American women now have the lowest breastfeeding rates in the country.

Slavery

Before Blacks were brought to America, they enjoyed all the freedom that life had to offer their culture. Parenting was a village, or community, effort.

Fathers were charged to rear up their sons as men. Mothers were a primary part of African life. They took care of the village – cooking, nurturing the children, tending to and cultivating the gardens, and other duties. An African woman became pregnant, gave birth, and breastfed. Childbirth was a rite of passage for African women. Young women were esteemed when they became mothers. Motherhood was revered.

Breastfeeding was an extension of mothering. It was a part of the birth continuum. There were no infant formula representatives peddling their wares through the African villages. There was not a single breastmilk substitute. Breastfeeding was the norm.

Breastmilk was considered a powerful indicator of luck. If a woman had an abundant and flowing milk supply, she was thought to be blessed and enjoyed all the privileges that revered motherhood offered from the village. On the other hand, when a mother had a limited milk supply, she was deemed cursed.

The choice to breastfeed in the African-American community goes deeper than simply what's best for baby. There's an old saying, "You must know your past to know your future." The same holds true with breastfeeding and African-American women. It's important to understand about our breastfeeding past to get a better understanding of our current state of breastfeeding, which may lead to a greater acceptance of breastfeeding in the future.

In Africa

Breastfeeding dates back to the beginning of man in Africa. From the earliest recordings of man, it's obvious that babies were fed breastmilk. We know that babies *had* to be breastfed since breastmilk substitutes – infant formula – did not exist. These early references about infant feeding practices were often in the form of pictures, hieroglyphics, and sculptures. You can walk into almost any museum and find art and sculptures from Ancient Egypt and other eras in African history that depict mothers with their baby latched onto the breast. They did not have the luxury of today's slings or nursing attire. Archeologists found the tomb of King Tut's wet nurse, which depicted the King sitting in the lap of Maya, his wet nurse. In ancient times, breastfeeding was generally written about in religious text. This is where we find the bulk of our information from early human history about breastfeeding.

The Holy Bible discusses breastfeeding as the normal manner of feeding a baby. A few stories highlighting this are found early on in the Bible. Sarah nursed her son for two years. Hannah promised that if God gave her a baby in her old age, she'd dedicate him to God. When he was born, before handing him over to God, she nursed him for an estimated two years. Many may be more familiar with the story of Moses. His mother had to hide him because Pharaoh wanted all Hebrew babies killed. So, she placed him in a basket and sent him down the river towards Pharaoh. Pharaoh's sister, who did not know he was Hebrew, found him and wanted to keep him as her own. But first, she sent him to a wet nurse for breastfeeding for an estimated two years. This shows the importance of breastmilk, even in ancient Egypt. There was no commercial infant formulas back then, so breastmilk was highly important for infant survival.

A wet nurse is a woman who breastfeeds a baby who is not her own. Wet nursing dates back to ancient societies. Then, wet nurses were used by women of stature and riches. It was an actual profession. There is even some evidence of an early, simplistic apparatus used to pump milk from a mother's breasts. In one tomb, a baby was found alongside what looked like a bottle. This is evidence – along with the Pyramids and their contribution to science and mathematics – that the early Egyptians were visionaries. Here, they were inventive in their view of breastfeeding and the freedom of mothers. At that time, however, the freedom of mothers was probably more related to upper class women who, while committed to pregnancy and childbirth, were busy ruling and/or being seen on a pedestal. Women nursed for at least three years.

Wet nursing was a regular part of life for non-royal Egyptian women, and those in other parts of Africa as well. For them, nursing another's baby was a functional matter, especially in the case of a mother's inability to produce milk, illness, or even death. Breastmilk was so important that babies were fed breastmilk from their mother, and often that of other women in the family group or tribe.

It's evident that herbs and other concoctions were medicinal. Fenugreek, often used today to help women increase their milk supply, is an ancient herb that has been used to treat a host of illnesses, particularly for women. It's likely that women used this herb, or another, thousands of years ago to help with their milk supply.

It's unfortunate that there is such a void of solid evidence about breastfeeding practices during the early part of our history. Breastfeeding research did not become an area of interest until the early part of the 1900's. Even then, it was not necessarily breastfeeding facts or problems that were of concern. It was not that breastfeeding rates were decreasing. The medical community began to take interest because of the increase in the research and manufacture of breastmilk substitutes, as well as an increase in infant health, illness, mortality, and a host of other issues facing women and the larger society.

Perhaps the most profound evidence about the exclusivity of breastfeeding during the early part of our history is the actual lack of information on the subject. We can assume that because breastfeeding was such a normal, daily part of a mother's existence (let's face it, there was no infant formula then) that there was no need to discuss it, write about it in documents, inscribe it in stone, paint it, or mold sculptures about it. Think about this for a minute. Historical records from early human history (which took place initially in Africa) generally highlight major issues, such as war, food, disease, land, exploration, religion, ancient "technology," and relationships. Ordinary nuances, such as hygiene, pregnancy, weight, and nail care were not usually historicized. We can guess by looking at other areas of life that people washed themselves, delivered babies, gained or lost weight, and took care of their nails in some fashion. Actually, as with much of our early history, women's experiences and issues are minimally mentioned. Stories were often handed down through oral traditions, through families. It was rarely written. The fact that breastfeeding is not often written about during that part of history, but clearly shown in art, indicates that breastfeeding was done exclusively and was vital, to the point of hiring wet nurses when a mother was unable or refused to breastfeed.

During Slavery

Breastfeeding has been part of the African culture for thousands of years. To date, there is little evidence of any breastmilk substitutes in early African history. Breastfeeding was a normal part of life. Wet nursing was also normal, and an essential part of daily life. Weaning tended to happen anywhere from two to five years of age in Ancient Egypt, and up to six years in some tribal groups in East Africa. Breastfeeding was a tradition that African women sustained consistently through European invasion and the subsequent slave trade. Please note that while this is not meant to be a lesson on slavery, it's vital for us to look at certain areas of this time in history because it sheds light on the breakdown in our breastfeeding tradition.

Europeans began their domination and devastation of the African continent and her people around the 1400's. By the time the slave trade began to flourish between Africa, America, and the Caribbean islands, millions upon millions of African families were broken apart. During the Middle Passage, the time and voyage from the African continent to its final slave port in one of the three major destinations, an estimated six million Africans died on board those ships. Conditions were inhumane. Africans from different regions, speaking different languages, and living different cultural traditions, were packed like cargo in the hull of the ship. For the months-long journey it took to reach the slave ports, they were rarely allowed on the deck. This means they did not receive fresh air or the sunlight that was a part of all African culture. They were fed slop, and the little water they received was polluted and transmitted infections and disease of the sort the Africans had not been exposed to. They were not allowed to wash or to expel human waste in a sanitary manner. Eating, sleeping, and expelling fecal waste was all done in the same location. Many died from the contamination and illnesses this type of environment created. Still others died from suicide. If ever allowed on deck, many attempted to throw themselves into the ocean.

If a suicide attempt failed, the slave was brutally beaten as an example of what would happen if others attempted to kill themselves.

As you can imagine, many women lost their lives. Pregnant women were forced to give birth to their babies in the same place they expelled bodily waste. Thousands of babies died, while many mothers killed their babies to protect them from such a cruel fate. Mothers did breastfeed the babies who survived during the Middle Passage. This was obviously the only way babies survived those months at sea. It was one African tradition, one way of life that could not be stripped from them. Breastfeeding was likely the only comfort African women had through the passage to a new land. Further, breastfeeding and breastmilk were likely the only comfort for a newborn, baby, and toddler. Imagine a newborn being too hot or feverish, locked in the hull of a ship? His body temperature could be balanced or regulated by breastfeeding. What about a baby facing growth spurts during the journey? Breastmilk could be produced to the point of satiating and filling his needs. And how about the foreign diseases and other illnesses the baby or toddler was exposed to? Breastmilk provided the only protection for the health of the child. And the African women who gave birth on the ships? Breastfeeding helped to stop postpartum bleeding, which surely would have led to infection and ultimately death. The Middle Passage is undoubtedly one of the most horrible times in the history of our people; yet, through the natural and age-old act of breastfeeding, lives were saved at a time when life, and God, were all our people had.

Once slaves arrived in America or on one of the Caribbean islands, conditions were far from improved. Families were separated, tribes were scattered, and abuse continued. Women were beaten, fondled, raped, and forced onto public display. Mothers with breastfeeding young were lucky if they were allowed to stay together. African women undoubtedly had to breastfeed babies who were not their own since more families were broken than were allowed to stay together. During the early years of the slave trade and colonization, the African was almost completely stripped of any power. The main source of power the African woman had was belief in her god. She held onto her African spiritual traditions to keep her grounded and believing that life would turn out better for her family, her children. This was her strength. A main source of power the African woman had as a mother was breastfeeding, a vital characteristic that kept her innate sense of mothering intact, even to the extension of nursing babies who were not her own – African babies from other tribes. Even through the shock of culture disruption, language barriers, and an entirely new land, African women maintained the physical and emotional need to breastfeed their young.

On plantations, reproduction rights and all things maternal – care of children, decisions about child rearing – were stripped from the African slave. Her ability and decision to reproduce was under the rule and domain of the slave master. She could not decide when to have children or the number of children she wanted, nor could she make any decisions related to infant feeding. She could no longer participate in the selection of a husband, as she may have done in Africa. She was not prepared for mothering and marriage with traditional rituals and female rights of passage. The very part of her that made her a distinct person – her femininity – was not under her control.

Marriage among slaves was forbidden, in fact, illegal, without the prior knowledge and consent of the slave master. More often than not, slaves were not allowed to marry. They were, however, forced to mate, breed, and reproduce with whomever the slave master chose. He selected which man and woman would be together. His decision was not based on love or compatibility. It was based on the product of two strong slaves, which would mean offspring that would add to slave labor. By controlling marriage and male/female relationships, not to mention breaking up families and selling children to other plantations, the slave master could control slave behavior. Since families were broken and relationships selected by him, he could keep slave revolts, escape, and uprisings to a minimum.

With so much change within the slave community, family was not life-long. It was often brief and fleeting. Women had no choice in this area. Slave women were forced to have sex with multiple slave men over the years, at the choice and whim of her slave master. To defy this would mean a brutal or sometimes deadly beating. The same punishment would be rendered if the slave master found that she had planned a pregnancy.

Slave women either worked in the slave master's (main) house or in the field. Neither placement was better or worse than the other. Both slaves' lives revolved around the slave master, his wife (mistress of the house), and their children. The house slave's life included many dimensions. She:

- Lived in the main house and slept under the bed of the mistress or with the children.

- Was on duty 24 hours a day.

- Cooked, tended the chickens and cows.

- Cleaned the main house.

- Made, mended, and washed clothes.

- Cared for minor medical issues within the main house.

- Was the personal maid of the mistress. She washed and styled the mistress' hair, helped her dress, took care of any of the mistress's personal needs and wants, and delivered her babies.

- Nurtured, disciplined, and played with the mistress' children.

- Breastfed/wet nursed the mistress' children.

The slave woman who worked in the field:

- Was in the field before the sun came up and left the field long after the sun set.

- Performed hard labor, including the cultivation of cotton, rice, corn, sugar, silk, and indigo.

- Planted and harvested crops and took care of farm animals.

- Managed the slave housing, including cooking, cleaning, washing, making and mending clothes, and caring for and breastfeeding the children.

These tasks were physically and mentally exhausting, particularly in the area of nurturing. On top of the backbreaking, labor-intensive lifestyle of the slave women, she habitually had to not just nurture and take care of the needs of the slave master's children, but she also had to give them life with her breastmilk, generally for up to two years. It's ironic that slave women were considered savage and not worthy of any human rights, yet her milk was good enough to nourish the slave master's children. She was believed to be unfit for living a dignified life in society and expressing the human emotion of love, but her breasts were desired for the important, life-giving task of breastfeeding. It's obvious that even breastmilk was a commodity for the benefit of the slave master and his plantation.

There is no doubt about the close bond that breastfeeding creates between a mother and child, or a woman and a baby. It's only natural then, that the slave women and the slave master's children would develop close bonds that lasted into adulthood. In spite of that, irony rears its head again in the fact that the very babies the slave woman nursed and cared for, would later become the cruel owner that enslaved her.

What about her own children? Was she allowed to nurse them? The only reason slave women were allowed to breastfeed was that it was free food for the baby, and it reduced the cost of feeding another slave. It was not because the slave master had a warm and fuzzy feeling about the importance of breastfeeding or that he wanted to give the slave woman some reprieve to relax from her hard labor. No, it was all a part of the carefully orchestrated life of the slave to better yield success in the increased production of slaves for labor.

The slave woman couldn't breastfeed on demand, as is important for the health of any newborn. She only had one day "free" of her slave duties. This was the day she gave birth. She returned to work the day after giving birth! She usually had less than 24 hours to spend bonding with and breastfeeding her baby. She could only nurse her baby, generally, two to three times a day. If she were lucky, she was allowed to carry the baby with her in the fields, which allowed her to nurse while she worked. This only lasted for a short period of time, probably a matter of weeks. Breastfeeding while working was physically challenging, as she was already on her feet the entire day. This regulated breastfeeding yielded many, many unhealthy babies whose growth was underdeveloped, yielding a generation of short slaves. The slave woman's diet, work load, and regulated feedings led to high infant mortality in the slave quarters. Most plantations allowed slaves to eat two to three times a day. Slaves lived on a meager and unwholesome diet of rationed cornmeal, pork, and molasses. They rarely received fresh meat, fruit, and vegetables. This poor diet, added to long hours of work, and less than seven hours of sleep a night often led to a poor quality and quantity of breastmilk in the slave woman – especially those who worked in the field. The above mix of poor diet and long, laborious work days worked to reduce the progesterone levels in a pregnant woman's body, which is a key hormone in getting a woman's breasts ready for breastfeeding.

Slave women were forced to feed their young regular food much too soon since their breastfeeding's were controlled by the slave master. Infants were given a mixture of cow's milk, cornbread, molasses, and the liquid from cooked greens. We know now that almost 100% of the African-American population is lactose intolerant (unable to digest the lactose/sugar found in milk.) The cow's milk used was often toxic and full of pollutants. If milk was not used, then contaminated water (slaves did not have access to natural or clean water) replaced it. This "food" was devoid of the proper amount of vitamins, minerals, proteins, and antibodies vital for an infant. This early introduction of solid food, although not quite as early as days after birth, is still a part of the African-American culture today. Again, there was a high rate of infant mortality because of disease and starvation. High infant mortality was not a priority for slave masters. They were more concerned about increasing numbers. If infants were dying, they just increased the pregnancies of the slave women.

Weaning tended to happen between nine and 12 months. Some weaning occurred within months if the mother's milk was of poor quality. Since breastfeeding is a natural form of birth control when feedings are not interrupted, child spacing can be optimal. However, many slave-owners deliberately shortened a slave woman's lactation, so she could get pregnant again and deliver more slave labor. Infants who still needed breastmilk were sent to a wet nurse (a slave, of course) whose sole job may have been breastfeeding the slaves' and slave master's children. Thousands of slave women died during or soon after childbirth because of malnutrition and the effects of hard labor on pregnancy – not to mention a lack of prenatal care. This again led to the neglect of breastfed infants. Early weaning was particularly harmful for the slave infant because of the unsanitary, infectious conditions associated with living in slave quarters.

The slave woman was considered a breeder, an important component of the slave master's livestock. His goal for her was to give birth to as many babies as possible, which would ultimately lead to more slave labor, a commodity during slavery. Her main responsibility was to reproduce. The average age for a slave woman to give birth was in her teens. It was not unusual for a slave woman to give birth to up to 15 babies or more; yet she may have had a large number of miscarriages. Slave women who delivered many babies were considered "good breeders" for the slave master. She tended to have longevity on a plantation, whereas slave women who could not yield a large number of babies were sold quickly. Once a slave girl reached adolescence and childbearing age, she became of interest to the slave master for her breeding ability and sexuality.

Slave women of all ages were easy prey for slave masters. She ultimately became the "other woman" and birthed a generation of bi-racial slave children. These children, early in slavery, were treated just like the rest of the slaves, working in the fields or in the main house. The slave woman raped for his sexual pleasure was certainly not treated any different. Later, when slavery began to weaken, they were given some privileges or freedom. Imagine, for a moment, the emotional and psychological effect of giving birth to your slave master's children, breastfeeding them, all the while breastfeeding the children of your mistress and slave master.

At this point in our history, breastfeeding had begun its slow demise in our community. Slavery redefined breastfeeding. For us, breastfeeding was once a traditional, normal part of being a mother. Breastfeeding was an extension of pregnancy and childbirth. It was a necessity that involved the love and care of our babies, with weaning around age three. We came to America with this tradition intact. Once reaching these shores, breastfeeding began to deviate from being an act of love to an association with the brutality of the slave experience. Breastfeeding our own was no longer in our control because breastfeeding of the slave master's babies took precedence. The formative breastmilk substitute was milk of vegetable and greens' liquid and cornmeal.

Mothering and the slave woman had two dimensions: The external part, based on her condition in slavery, and the internal part, based on her mind and emotions. Superficially, on a very basic level, the slave woman's role as a mother was non-existent. She was a gateway for her child's birth, and nothing more. This was carefully orchestrated by the slave master to increase his human resources. As mentioned earlier, her sole duty was to do what the slave master required of her, including field work, reproduction, wet nursing, and sex. She could not choose when to breastfeed, when to start solids, how to care for a sick child, who the child would marry, where he/she could go or who they could play with, what the child would be when he/she grew up. Just as her basic rights as a human were stripped from her, so was her experience with mothering. The usual nurturing that is part of being a mother was not a part of the slave woman's experience. She worked long hours and had little time to spend with her children. She had, at best, brief moments in the morning, before work, and at night, after work, to focus on mothering.

The mother-child bond that is critical for emotional healing for women and psychological development for children was almost non-existent. During this time, however, white mothers lived a life full of the bonding and nurturing that is essential to mothering. They had the option, and often chose, however, to turn over nurturing, breastfeeding, and childcare to the slave woman at will.

Internally, the slave woman's spirit was extraordinary – resilience of stone. Few figures in history can be examined and proved to be as resilient. On the outside, her conditions were merciless; yet inside, she held onto some hope that she would make it and her race would, also. This is evident in the legacy she left in the product of her sweat and physical labor – agricultural development and architectural foundations upon which this country was built – as well as the life she gave to thousands of Black and White babies through her breastmilk.

Breastfeeding was likely the only link to a slave woman's mothering experience. Breastfeeding her baby was the last link to mothering because she was not allowed to make decisions about any aspect of her child's life. Breastfeeding was the slave woman's only means of empowerment since every aspect of her life was tightly regulated. It was often all the slave woman could ever do for her baby, since the slave babies often died young or were sold to other plantations, never to be reunited with their mother. Breastfeeding was often a final link between a slave woman and her child.

Toni Morrison's Pulitzer Prize winner, *Beloved* (2006), illustrates a vivid, fictional example – based on a historical figure – of the psychological impact of *not* being able to breastfeed on slave women. The main character, Seth, lives a large portion of her life in deep despair over not being able to breastfeed her babies, which was the only link to motherhood and nurturing she had as a slave. On top of that, the slave master's nephews abused her and drank the milk from her breasts that could not be provided to her own baby. Breastmilk is woven throughout *Beloved* to show the emotional impact of a slave woman's inability to nurture and mother her young.

Post Slavery

Breastfeeding was a traditional part of the African mother's everyday life. It was a culturally acceptable part of African life. Breastfeeding was not just part of tradition. It was also considered a spiritual act. Women who produced milk and nourished their babies were considered blessed, while those who could not produce breastmilk were considered cursed. Ancient Egyptians wrote about and carved statues with depictions of breastfeeding. Tribal religions and belief in gods also speak to the importance of breastfeeding. The Bible, the Koran, and other religious texts that African women were guided by reinforced the spiritual act of breastfeeding. Breastmilk was believed to have special powers, and was even used to bring peace between warring groups. Slave women brought the tradition of breastfeeding to America and continued to breastfeed their own children, and wet-nursed countless others, throughout slavery, and afterwards.

Breastfeeding was, however, no longer solely associated with mothering and bonding. It began to take on a new twist. Breastfeeding was connected to slavery, abuse, and meeting the needs of the captor's children over that of our own. Even with our rich cultural heritage in this area, breastfeeding for us was infected with the psychological and emotional affects of slavery. After over 250 years of brutality, slavery "officially" ended in 1863, with most slaves not set free until years later. For many years, slavery was against the law, but it was still practiced, especially in the south. Even after the Civil War ended and slaves were freed in large numbers, their plight was still dreadful.

A small victory of freedom was the regaining of some control over their lives, particularly in the area of marriage and childbirth. Family was once again a true part of our frame of reference and familial roots could be planted. Yet, this was short-lived, as racism was still an epidemic that plagued our community. And, with larger societal problems – World Wars – the family took another hit. We moved from finally having two parents in the home to one or both parents leaving to find work. Money was difficult to earn, so parents had to go to the North during the Great Migration or back to sharecropping for months at a time to provide for their families. Black babies were left in the care of older family members. African-American babies were forced, once again, to take breastmilk substitutes that were nutritionally unsafe and devoid of antibodies – leading to increased Black infant mortality. Once again, breastfeeding rates were lowered because babies were separated from their mothers due to continued and heightened societal factors, work, family separation, and wet-nursing.

Many African-American women worked the same types of positions they held during slavery, with the exception of being free. Wet nursing was still a part of her frame of reference in the early part of the 1900's. The pay for this type of position was deplorable. In 1912, the *Indecent* newspaper quoted a 40-year-old Black nurse as saying, "Perhaps a million of us are introduced daily to the privacy of a million chambers throughout the South, and hold in our arms a million white children, thousands of whom, as infants, are suckled at our breasts – during my lifetime I myself have served as "wet nurse" to more than a dozen white children. In the distant future, it may be, centuries and centuries hence, a monument of brass or stone will be erected to the Old Black Mammies of the South, but what we need is present help, present sympathy, better wages, better hours, more protection, and a chance to breathe for once while alive as free women. If none others will help us, it would seem that the Southern white women themselves might do so in their own defense, because we are rearing their children – we feed them, we bathe them, we teach them to speak the English language, and in numberless instances we sleep with them – and it is inevitable that the lives of their children will in some measure be pure or impure according as they are affected by contact with their colored nurses."

She mentioned later in the article that her 13-year-old daughter was employed as a wet nurse and paid $1.50 a week. Wet nursing was a profession that goes back to ancient times. After slavery ended, most women employed as wet nurses were Black, or some poorer White women. Wealthy women and physicians hired wet nurses because of their support of the vital importance of breastmilk for an infant's health. During this time, the breastmilk from wet nurses – who were largely African-American – was determined to be inadequate for White babies. Human milk banks accepted breastmilk from Blacks with reservations, once again, about its quality for White babies. It would appear that to the medical community and affluent White mothers, *breastmilk* was a commodity that was essential for health reasons, and had little to do with bonding and nurturing a baby. There seems to be a certain freedom that White mothers desired during the early part of the 20th century.

The late 19th and early 20th centuries also brought new advancements in medical technology. There was a shift from homebirths and midwives to more hospital-based deliveries, medications during labor, and infant formula use. Physicians began to discourage the use of wet nurses and midwifery services. Up to that time, all births – for Black and White women – happened at home. Black women were assisted either by a sister, mother, friend, or the "woman who caught babies." Today, she'd be called a midwife. Hospital births were generally considered by the public as unsanitary. Women who delivered in hospitals were women from low-economic groups and were given free services, and chiefly acted as guinea pigs for the medical profession. By the 1930's, the practice of midwifery and home births was in the minority, and hospital births became the norm. The late 19th century brought with it two drugs to ease the pain of childbirth. Many women were routinely put to sleep during childbirth, and those drugs have advanced a widespread use of a variety of pain relievers during childbirth today. With the increase in the popularity of hospital births came another method for capitalism. Fees for hospital births pushed many low-income women out of this practice because services were no longer offered for free. Many Black women, especially those in southern and more country areas still had births at home. With hospital births came new practices in infant care, including separation of mother from baby, which can inhibit breastfeeding success.

While advances were being made in the area of hospital birthing practices, which aided in our deviation from traditional practices, breastmilk's greatest nemesis stepped onto the world scene. Artificial breastmilk, infant formula, or whatever you'd like to call it — a new product was being developed. One of the first companies to create a safer cow's milk blend was the Walker-Gordon Milk Laboratory. They created a "formula," method, recipe, to make cow's milk more acceptable to an infant's system. Even as early as the 1890's, the company was distributing their product to mothers. In less than 10 years, there were Walker-Gordon Milk laboratories in 10 cities across the country. More than 20 types of infant formula were produced during the late 1890's. Dairy pasteurization and safe milk storage was still a problem. Early formula did not have quality measures for safe storage, which led to frequent contamination. Many of these formulas were of the powder type, which had to be mixed with water. At this time, public sanitation and safe water was a major health concern. Often, formula was mixed with unsafe water, leaving a baby open to disease. Formula wasn't fortified with iron until later. Bottles were not yet safe, and adequate sterilization was frequently a problem. Many people made infant formula at home because commercial formulas were only affordable to the wealthy. This homemade formula consisted of a can of condensed milk (Carnation or Pet), water, and corn syrup (Karo). This practice was especially common in the African-American community through the 1950's.

Physicians and formula manufacturers worked hard in the early to mid 1900's to create an infant formula that emulated the nutrients found in breastmilk. The fact that a breastmilk substitute was based on the milk of another species, the cow, and was created in a scientific lab is rather scary. The physicians were concerned about perfecting their product, not the health of the infants who would consume the formula. They made many, many attempts and scientific experiments to duplicate the composition of breastmilk. Unfortunately, at the time, the components of breastmilk were still a phenomenon to the medical community. A wide variety of formula was manufactured by different scientists, trying to get it right. By the 1950's, there was such a demand for infant formula that manufacturers created a prepared, concentrated formula with reduced cost, so the product could reach the most people. The correlation between the increased mass production of infant formula, the decline in breastfeeding rates, and the increased infant mortality is evident.

Early 20th Century

Breastfeeding rates and statistics did not begin to be measured until the early 1900's. The studies largely focus on infant mortality and not the reduction of breastfeeding. Few studies are found even then. But in the early 1900s, more White mothers exclusively breastfed than Black mothers, and more Black mothers than White mothers were breastfeeding and supplementing.

Today

The breastfeeding rates of African-American women today are the sum total of experience with slavery, racism, economics, breakdown of the family, and limited access to breastfeeding resources, education, and support. In recent history and at present, African-American women have some of the lowest breastfeeding rates in the country. Up to the turn of the century in the early 1900's, our breastfeeding rates were higher than today. This is largely due to the last remnants of the breastfeeding tradition we held onto, along with the lack of adequate breastmilk substitutes available to us.

Guiding Principle: Respect the history and culture of breastfeeding for African-Americans and how it affects their lactation practices.

Chapter Three.
Barriers to Breastfeeding – Initiation/Duration

Due to the barriers that Black women face, both internal (perceived myths, lack of confidence, doing something different than others in her circle, etc.), and external (cultural stigma, lack of support, excessive marketing by infant formula companies in the community, lack of education from medical professionals, lack of Black IBCLCs, etc.), Black women either don't breastfeed or breastfeed for an exceedingly shorter period of time than other mothers.

The Lactation Landscape

The major trends that African-American women face fall into five main areas:

1. Low initiation and duration of breastfeeding

2. Infant formula marketing

3. Lack of normalcy

4. Strong belief in breastfeeding myths

5. Lack of effective breastfeeding education and promotion

The first trend will be discussed below. The other trends will be discussed in subsequent chapters.

Low Initiation and Duration of Breastfeeding

Initiation and duration of breastfeeding in the Black community is a lesson in peeling back many layers, many of which will be reviewed in the following chapters. The decision to breastfeed in this community is compounded uniquely and overwhelmingly because of the following factors:

- A general belief in the importance of breastfeeding.

- Seeing breastfeeding models in one's family.

- A conviction that one will breastfeed, no matter the barriers or trouble faced during the experience.

- Lack of support by family, who face the same barriers.

- Lack of support by husbands and boyfriends who do not understand the importance of breastfeeding.

Support

The choice to breastfeed for an African-American woman comes with thoughts about how best to feed her baby, but also with concerns about "how do I actually do this?" Since breastfeeding has not been a part of the African-American culture for many generations, many who choose to do so are the first in years in her family. Modeling of breastfeeding behavior will often start with today's Black mom. Her peers are more likely to support her than family members, who did not breastfeed.

La Leche League International (LLLI) has been the primary organization that supports women who breastfeed, providing support groups, peer counselors, literature, training courses, conferences, advocacy, and groundbreaking change in the field of mother-to-mother support. LLLI understands, as does everyone in the lactation field, how vital it is for mothers to have support readily available during the lactation years.

Organizations like LLLI, however, have not made much progress in providing support to African-American women. It's not intentional. The dynamic of how they've functioned over the years have not met the needs of the average Black mom. Most mother-to-mother support groups meet during the day when Black women are working, or are held outside of African-American communities.

Since 2000, there has been some success with groups that have focused on providing mothering and lactation support to Black moms. Organizations like the African American Breastfeeding Alliance (AABA), The Black Mother's Breastfeeding Association (BMBA), Soul Food for Your Baby (SFFYB), and others have worked diligently to promote breastfeeding to the Black community, in addition to providing various means of support to the women who choose to breastfeed. Projects have included workshops to educate healthcare professionals about working with the African-American community, breastfeeding classes for moms, mothering/breastfeeding support groups, and marketing campaigns to reach more Black moms. Efforts have been growing, yet frequently are inhibited due to lack of sustainable funding.

Economics

Older, more educated African-American women who earn a higher income are more likely to breastfeed. Younger, less educated African-American women who earn a low income, or who receive government assistance, are less likely to breastfeed. While African-American women in general are less likely to breastfeed than other races, education and economic status gives more access to resources.

Quality prenatal care and stable health insurance are standard practice for Black women who earn middle to higher incomes. Paying for breastfeeding classes, a Lactation Consultant's services, and purchasing an effective double electric breast pump is not unusual to this mom. The ability, or choice, to continue breastfeeding upon return to work or the ability to stay at home for an extended period of time to raise a baby may even be a possibility – no matter how remote.

What's interesting to note here is that Black women who receive quality prenatal care tend to have the same birth outcomes as Black women who receive inadequate or no prenatal care as documented in a PBS special (*When the Bough Breaks* http://www.pbs.org/unnaturalcauses/hour_02. htm) that followed the lives of African-American women from polar different backgrounds – economics, environment, background, education.

Oddly, Black women who are more educated and make more money tend to have worse birth outcomes. The research found that racism and employment discrimination are the prime factors that lead to high rates of preterm births, low birthweight babies, infant mortality, poor birth outcomes, and poor maternal health. Ultimately, it would follow that breastfeeding rates would be lacking as well.

Return to Work

A key barrier to the initiation and/or continuation of breastfeeding among African-American women is the belief that breastfeeding must stop upon return to work. This barrier is due to the lack of prenatal breastfeeding education and postnatal breastfeeding support (more below), and uncertainty about how pumping will fit into the scope of employment and day-to-day living.

When you look at the breastfeeding rates of Black women and see the severe decline after initiation to six months, the issue of returning to work is evident. Most African-American women return to work at six weeks, the normal maternal leave policy in the U.S. Some take additional time with the Family Medical Leave Act, which may extend her time at home with her child up to twelve weeks. Unfortunately, the majority of African-American women in the workforce return to work early and have given up breastfeeding because:

- She has not been educated about the importance of continuing to breastfeed after the early prenatal period.

- She believes her breastmilk is not sufficient to meet the needs of a growing infant.

- She's concerned that her workplace will not accommodate time for pumping and/or private space.

- She cannot afford a double electric breast pump.

- She has already spent extra time caring for a sick baby in the NICU (remember Black babies have poor infant health outcomes) and fears asking for "extra" support from her employer.

- She does not have a supportive childcare provider who feels comfortable handling expressed breastmilk.

These are all very real barriers that African-American women face when it comes to deciding whether to continue breastfeeding after returning to work. Without support, planning, and preparation, the breastfeeding experience tends to be short-lived.

Chapter Four.
Barriers to Breastfeeding – Infant Formula Marketing

It is well documented that breastfeeding in the U.S. is not the standard method of infant feeding. In the African-American population, rates are far less than in other races. One of the foremost barriers to breastfeeding for Black mothers is the advertising of infant formula in this community. Infant formula is at least a $2 billion a year industry, with the inclusion of their subsidiary products, including bottles, nipples, infant water, pacifiers, infant vitamin supplements, infant colic drops, infant food, and a host of other baby products.

Infant formula companies have a monopoly on infant feeding – yes they make money on how we feed our babies. Breastmilk does not earn capital, so these companies earn money from supporting pregnancy magazines and many other products on the general consumer market (i.e. Nestle). When women read these magazines, the effective marketing leads them directly to the formula aisle, or at the very least, it takes away an openness to breastfeed.

When an African-American woman goes to her first doctor's visit, be she well-educated and have a medium to high income, or low income and less educated, she is given a diaper bag full of infant formula samples. How is this a barrier to breastfeeding? How is a bag of infant formula samples so impactful to African-American moms?

Marketing is defined as *the provision of goods or services to meet customer or consumer needs.* These diaper bags are an effective marketing tool: At first glance giving mom everything she needs to start taking care of her baby. The typical bag includes a sample of infant formula, diapers, wipes, a pregnancy health magazine, and coupons for more formula. Most women will then sign up for a free year's subscription to a parenting magazine and receive advertisements via snail and email for infant formula. Cases of infant formula may even be delivered during the pregnancy and after delivery. Months after the baby is born, mothers still receive coupons, samples, and other products from infant formula companies that "grow with the baby," further implanting the idea that infant formula is essential. WIC is the largest purchaser of infant formula, and many Black women receive WIC benefits. Hence, infant formula's marketing reaches African-American mothers at a higher rate than other races.

If the Black mother is a participant in the WIC Program, the marketing of infant formula is built into the services she receives. She will receive supplementary free infant formula for her baby, and other free food until her child is five years old. While WIC agencies are federally mandated to provide breastfeeding education and programs to participants, it is one of the largest purchasers of infant formula in the world. WIC's commitment to providing breastfeeding support is regional, certainly not national. Recently WIC agencies across the country were given millions of dollars to enhance their peer counselor programs. Unfortunately, while federally mandated to be used for breastfeeding promotion, these funds seldom met the targeted need.

The effective marketing of infant formula has created a belief in the African-American community that infant formula is just as good as breastmilk for infant feeding. This belief has been a key problem in breastfeeding promotion efforts. There is a major divide between formula company marketing dollars, and those "marketing" breastfeeding. With millions spent on infant formula, these companies have seemingly infinite amounts of money to pour into reaching their target audience: Black mothers who would otherwise choose to breastfeed.

Chapter Five.
Lack of Normalcy

Chances are you are reading this book because breastfeeding is no longer the norm in the African-American community in your area, and you want to know why and what you can do to make a difference. Breastfeeding is not a norm in this community, as it is in most other racial groups, based on a number of factors, largely historical ones:

- Slavery

- Breakdown of the African-American family due to history

- Banishment from the career of wet-nursing

- Death of midwifery

- Lack of healthcare access

- Switch from home births to hospital delivery and care

- Infant formula and marketing to Black families

Since breastfeeding was once a cultural norm for Africans, and then African-Americans up until the early 1900's, it would follow that historical situations, largely outside of their control, began to change such a traditional behavior. This cultural shift in infant nutrition and maternal practice was slow, subliminal, and subtly ingrained in such a way that today a previous tradition, or norm, is long forgotten.

Support of Family and Friends

Studies have shown, particularly research done by Dr. Yvonne Bronner and colleagues at Johns Hopkins University and others, that the African-American woman's infant feeding choices and breastfeeding habits are highly influenced by their husbands, male counterparts, mothers, female family members, and friends. OB/GYNs, nurses, and other healthcare professionals don't have the influence that family members have on this group's decision to breastfeed: The family does (Bentley et al., 1999; Wolfberg et al, 2004).

Since African-Americans have not breastfed, have had the lowest breastfeeding rates for generations, and breastfeeding has not been a traditional part of the culture for even longer, the breastfeeding connection across the Black community has been largely broken. As I've said throughout this book, history, barriers, myths, and lack of education have played a role in the breastfeeding disparity in the African-American community. This has not just affected the Black mom, but breastfeeding beliefs in the entire race.

African-American mothers' infant feeding choices are greatly influenced by her family history. If she is from a family with a history of formula feeding, then nine times out of ten, she will choose to formula feed. Since formula is the infant food of choice today, most Black women are likely to feed their babies infant formula.

However, when Black women choose to breastfeed, they are rarely supported, unless it is a part of their family history and is modeled in their respective communities. If their husbands and partners support breastfeeding, then they will breastfeed. Conversely, if husbands/partners disregard, don't understand, and do not support breastfeeding, African-American women will either not even try breastfeeding, breastfeed for a short period of time, or supplement with infant formula.

It is vital to not only promote breastfeeding to and educate Black women, but also to extend this education to her entire family. Tips:

- Include your client's husband or partner in prenatal and breastfeeding classes.

- If there is no partner, include the mother or another family member/friend.

- Educate the husband, partner, and family on the benefits of breastfeeding.

- Always respect the male counterpart, whether they are married or not. This is vital, and is an institutional problem that is widespread in hospitals and other medical facilities.

- You will go far by asking directly for the family's support and help in encouraging and supporting breastfeeding.

Chapter Six.
Barriers to Breastfeeding – Strong Belief in Breastfeeding Myths

People often say, "Everyone believes in breastfeeding myths. What's so different about Black women?" The truth is that while we tend to *know* "breastmilk" is best, the deep belief in myths is not simply areas of discussion: these beliefs actually stop us from breastfeeding.

Breastfeeding Is Painful

For instance, the majority of Black women believe that breastfeeding IS painful. Professionals know that the information counter to this myth is broad, but breastfeeding support is copiously lacking in Black areas. When Black women try breastfeeding, many don't have lactation consultants or peer counselors available to help them through those first few weeks that are often challenging. If breastfeeding is done improperly, it entails a level of pain and the moms give up. When a negative experience occurs with breastfeeding in the Black community, it seems to spread like a plague that can't be contained. It goes viral and leads to misconceptions that stop, hinder, and reduce the initiation and duration of breastfeeding.

My Breastmilk Is Not Sufficient: Infant Formula Is as Good as Breastmilk

There is a far-reaching belief among African-American women that breastmilk (and formula for that matter, but breastmilk more so) is insufficient to sustain the nutritional needs of an infant. Early introduction of solid foods is endemic. Helping clients to understand the nutritive benefits of breastmilk is important. Further, tap into another angle – the adverse effects of infant formula.

African-American children have some of the highest rates of childhood obesity (DHHS Office of Minority Health, 2011). This has been deemed by some researchers to be partially due to early introduction of solid foods and lack of breastfeeding (Thompson & Bentley, 2012). African-American infants are regularly given solid foods as early as one to two weeks after birth, and at the latest, within the first month. This may include rice cereal mixed with infant formula, breastmilk, or water. Other foods and supplements given are mashed potatoes and gravy, fruit juices, and soda.

These solids are not always given directly by the African-American mother. They are more likely to be given by an older African-American grandmother, aunt, or caregiver, or by the mother on the advice of this older family sage. Introduction of solid foods before the first four months of life occurs across the board in the African-American community, regardless of education and socio-economic factors.

How do you combat these barriers? Educate. Educate. Educate.

- Do not always discuss the benefits of breastmilk. Instead talk about the insufficiency of infant formula.

- Educate families about the negative health impact of infant formula.

- Discuss nutrition and how the early introduction of solid foods is unhealthy and can cause all the health issues that they, the adult African Americans, are coping with – hypertension, diabetes, etc.

- Empower mothers to make infant feeding choices for themselves, regardless of opinions of family members: they have the power to choose for their babies.

- Remember to include that infant formula does not protect against disease – be sure to highlight asthma!

Chapter Seven.
Lack of Effective Breastfeeding Education and Promotion

Agency Promotion

Breastfeeding promotion in the African-American community began with a focus on the WIC (Women, Infants, and Children Program) population. Research in the 90's and government programs began to surface due to the findings that Black women were breastfeeding at markedly lower rates than White and Hispanic women. While the WIC Program, Health and Human Services Office on Women's Health Breastfeeding Campaign, and others sought to increase breastfeeding awareness, these programs only targeted women of low income and educational status. What about African-American women of middle and upper incomes, who have higher education? Those women were and still are left out of many of the targeted programs to promote breastfeeding in African-American communities. It's as if lower income Black women need more breastfeeding assistance than other Black women. In fact, across the board, Black women of all socioeconomic status have the same birth outcomes, and generally the same breastfeeding rates. It would follow that breastfeeding promotion should be spread to all African-American women, regardless of income or education.

The problem with many of these well-intentioned, researched, and organized education and promotion programs is two-fold. One, they don't get the buy-in of the audience they are trying to help – African-American mothers, and, of course, their families, too. This is a systematic government problem of going into communities with a plan that often collapses because the target group was not asked what their intrinsic problems are and what solutions they feel will best assist them. Breastfeeding promotion programs often use the approach from White and Hispanic communities without effective and specific cultural vetting to make promotion successful, as well as getting buy-in from Black moms. Black mothers know what they need; however, no one is asking what those needs are and how programs can be useful in meeting those breastfeeding needs. Two, breastfeeding education and promotion is generally tacked onto other programs, be it WIC, Healthy Start, Black Infant Health, or some other government program. Black women are multi-dimensional, and this insular approach at looking at Black women has been an enormous disservice to educate them about breastfeeding. There is absolutely zero need to start breastfeeding support groups by adding them onto WIC appointments or Healthy Start and government programs. The rare breastfeeding support group or education class specifically for Black women has come from groups like the African American Breastfeeding Alliance (AABA) and Mocha Moms (group for mothers of color). Breastfeeding education and promotion can and should be singular, not just add-ons to existing programs.

Education of Medical and Healthcare Professionals

Healthcare providers have been providing a disservice to pregnant and lactating Black women for far too long. Few Black women receive breastfeeding education during the prenatal period – the absolute critical time to educate Black women on breastfeeding. When Black women do receive breastfeeding education, it tends to be outside of the prenatal or physician's setting – a WIC clinic, Healthy Start, church group, or some social setting. Black women who are WIC participants tend to receive more breastfeeding education than those not on the program, depending on how breastfeeding supportive that agency is.

Doctors on a large scale do not provide lactation education (Cricco-Lizza, 2006). It's a broad sweeping assumption in the medical community – from the physician's office to the labor and delivery staff – that Black women won't breastfeed. This is due to our low breastfeeding rates and seeming aversion to breastfeeding. At any rate, since obstetricians and pediatricians receive minimal, if any, lactation education in medical school, they are not usually equipped to provide adequate breastfeeding education and support. The Academy of Breastfeeding Medicine has done a great deal of work to provide substantive lactation courses for doctors; however, these courses are not yet the norm. If medical professionals are not adequately, or at the very least, minimally trained in breastfeeding education and management, then Black women will continue to lag behind in breastfeeding rates.

Doctors are not the only members of the healthcare team whose lactation management skills are lacking. Nurses, including neonatal nurses and pediatric nurse practitioners, nutritionists, dieticians, healthcare staff, and the WIC team are all often behind the lactation education curve. Frequently, the childbirth educator, doula, midwife or breastfeeding peer counselor are the only professional that offers breastfeeding education, support, and/or asks the simple question, "Have you thought about how you will feed your new baby?" If a Black mom does not see one of these professionals during her pregnancy, or has not seen breastfeeding modeled in her family or community, she will time and again choose not to breastfeed.

What can you do to incorporate easy breastfeeding promotion during routine visits with your African-American clients?

- Use each prenatal visit to have a brief discussion about breastfeeding.
- Ask her how she feels about breastfeeding, what she knows about it.
- Discuss any fears, challenges she may have.
- Provide small bits of education about the how-to's.
- Dispel myths and discuss support.
- Be open about the urgent health implications for Black infant and maternal health – be graphic.

Guiding Principle: Develop useful methods to help clients overcome barriers.

Chapter Eight.
Lactation Counseling –
Communication

One of the most important aspects of lactation counseling among Black women is for the lactation professional to understand her role – to offer education and support. Often, problems arise between well-meaning lactation consultants and their Black clients due to the LC's overzealous commitment to breastfeeding, her agency/hospital's policies, or her judgments about the client's lifestyle or breastfeeding choices.

Some might ask, "What's different about breastfeeding for Black women?" If you add the state of Black infant health in America with low breastfeeding rates, it's apparent that there is a need to have a targeted approach to effectively reach and provide breastfeeding management to African-American women. Today's lactation consultant, breastfeeding peer counselor, nurse, doctor and other healthcare professional should be well versed in the cultural norms and nuances of the communities they serve. When it comes to lactation management and promotion, understanding the background of breastfeeding and African-Americans, and being as prepared as possible to communicate successfully, will take the encounter far.

What is Successful Lactation Counseling?

Is your bottom line to increase breastfeeding rates among your African-American clients? Has your agency signed onto the Surgeon General's *Call to Action on Breastfeeding* to reach underserved communities? Do you have to increase breastfeeding rates by 1%, 2%, or 5% in the coming year? Are your outreach goals designed to target African-American women in the WIC population and have them meet the Healthy People 2020 mandate set by the U.S. Department of Health and Human Services and the Centers for Disease Control?

What is your bottom line? What is your goal in lactation management and promotion among your Black clients?

The better, more successful approach is to ask, "What is my client's bottom line?" For far too long, well-meaning, hard-working lactation professionals have approached African-American women in the wrong way.

Frankly, when it comes to providing solutions to communities that are in a health disparate situation – as is the case with the low breastfeeding rates of Black women – professionals, government agencies, doctors, and others have used the wrong approach. To bring about effective, long-lasting change in any group, answers have to be vetted and approved by the group that "needs change." Answers are always more authentic when they are reached in an authentic manner.

What's In It For You?

When you change the lactation dial on your FM radio, are you tuning into WIFY – What's In It For You? Lactation professionals do a disservice to Black mothers by approaching their lactation experience just like all others. When Black women choose to breastfeed, wean early, supplement, or introduce solid foods early, it's not always about an aversion to breastfeeding. The history, cultural climate, internal and external barriers, belief in myths, and lifestyle she leads all mix together to create the Black woman you encounter in your lactation appointment, class, or event.

It's important to remind yourself of all it took for the African-American mom to meet you where you are in that moment. Ask yourself the following questions:

- What's in it for your African-American client?
- What's in it for the African-American baby?

Here are some African-American "isms" you may consider when communicating with your clients:

- Early introduction of solid foods
- Powerful breastfeeding advocates
- More likely to breastfeed if they are older and educated
- Kinship
- R-E-S-P-E-C-T
- DAD plays a vital role

When communicating with African-American women, give sample counseling dialogue scenarios and firmly establish the LC understands that the "bottom line" in breastfeeding lies with the mother, not the LC. Communication should also focus on members of the African-American woman's family and larger social group. Remember:

- Respect is fundamental.
- Be open and honest.
- Establish trust – don't sell dreams.
- Be professionally objective.

- Be flexible. You may not have the whole background for a woman's decision or push-back on a particular piece of advice. Listen closely and help her come to her own effective conclusions.

- Be direct. Don't beat around the bush. Don't sell dreams of breastfeeding grandeur.

- Conversational style is best. Condescending and "I'm the expert" attitudes don't work with breastfeeding management.

- Openly disagreeing is okay and works well with being direct, but remember to back it up with proper information.

- Eye contact is important.

- Less personal body space is okay. Sitting too close or touching without permission is a definite 'no-no.'

- Humor is good, but use with caution.

- Avoid euphemisms unless you are completely comfortable with them.

- Be yourself. Authenticity goes a long way.

- Understand cultural factors that lead to non-responsiveness and how culture impacts decision-making.

- Effective breastfeeding support is specific to the specific need. Keep it specific and not general.

- Be completely open and non-judgmental. Your background and goals are not relevant. Helping the mother is all that matters.

Guiding Principle: Develop a clear understanding of effective communication.

Chapter Nine.
Outshine Myths and Barriers through Counseling

Breastfeeding barriers and myths are the primary hurdles lactation professionals must cross to get African-American women to buy into breastfeeding. Each day, dedicated IBCLCs, breastfeeding peer counselors, labor and delivery nurses, midwives, doulas, and other members of the healthcare team seek creative ways to help Black mothers overcome these barriers.

How do you contend with early introduction of solid foods; cultural and family beliefs that undermine breastfeeding; lack of confidence in yourself, the practitioner, and the breastfeeding mother; and coping with lack of family/community support?

Educating yourself in advance about these special issues in the African-American community is your first step to being an effective lactation professional, as well as being equipped in advance with practical skills to help your clients.

The Lactation Professional's Role

Of my many years working to educate lactation professionals of different races on cultural competency, I've had to tow the line between brutal honesty and political correctness. It's been a fine dance between tempering feelings and being truthful about our differences, with a mix of true reality. The truth is there are about 95% White lactation consultants in this country, which means the odds of Black women working with an LC of color is rare.

Effective lactation care has been shown across the board and races to be most effective through peer-to-peer support. Not just peer counselor to client, peer to peer – as in people from the same community. In the area of breastfeeding, it's especially personal for Black women, with the history and challenges we've faced from tradition to disparate rates. Lactation professionals of color work particularly well in providing good and effectual breastfeeding care and management to Black women. However, due to the sheer lack of them in this country, the chance that Black women will have one is unlikely.

This is why non African-American lactation professionals want to know how to provide culturally specific care to their Black clients. Where does it start?

You, as the lactation professional, have to begin to search yourself and look within. You have to be truthful with yourself and answer the following questions – even journal about them. You'll be surprised at how revealing these answers can be.

- What's your personal style?

- How do you communicate?

- What have people told you about your ability to manage breastfeeding problems?

- Do you have preconceived beliefs about Black women and breastfeeding?

- Do you approach your African-American clients with the assumption that they won't breastfeed?

- What's your goal – a successful breastfeeding experience for the mom or increased breastfeeding rates?

- What's more important to you – getting the baby to the breast or what the Black mom wants/needs?

- How do you measure success in your practice or agency?

Lack of Confidence in Yourself as a Practitioner

Clients notice when you are uncomfortable about approaching them. Often, we act in two distinct ways when we are uncomfortable. One, we either overcompensate our abilities – act aggressively and overzealous, provide too much breastfeeding information, ignore mom's concerns, touch the mother without asking, and act on biased information. Or two, we don't show up out of fear of the unknown.

The best advice is to show up as yourself, with a clear mind that has explored all the questions in the previous section.

- Be yourself – you know You best.

- Don't use the same technique on each client – everyone is different.

- Listen. Listen. Listen. This calms the nerves and allows for your confidence to build.

- Do not try to be Who you think the client wants you to be – it's false and never works.

- Educate yourself on the plight of Black women and breastfeeding, and be ready for even more learning – knowledge is power.

- Recognize your own burnout. It is common in the lactation

profession and causes ineffective breastfeeding management, and sometimes inappropriate behavior or language.

Change the Language / Change the Approach

You can begin to use the following tips with the very next client you see. They are practical and will go a long way toward having a successful visit or educational/breastfeeding promotion experience with an African-American client.

- Remember RESPECT = an open door.

- Professional objectivity is important until trust and rapport is established.

- Understanding cultural factors can't be overstated.

- Practice nonjudgmental attitudes and behaviors – again this cannot be overstated.

- Recognize appropriate/inappropriate engagement – do not touch without asking.

- Don't patronize, pretend, sell dreams, or argue about breastfeeding – you will lose.

Guiding Principle: Develop useful methods to help clients overcome barriers.

Chapter Ten.
Helping Breastfeeding Mothers Return to Work

Being a stay-at-home mother has not historically been part of the African-American woman's experience.   More than 62% of African-American women work outside of their homes (Bureau of Labor and Statistics, 2012). That said the reality is that most African-American mothers have to return to the workplace during the standard maternity leave of six weeks. African-American teen mothers often have to return to school even earlier than that – sometimes as early as three weeks postpartum.

One of the leading barriers to breastfeeding in the African-American community is returning to work. Many African-American women will not initiate breastfeeding because they believe you can't continue breastfeeding after returning to work. Other African-American women will only commit to breastfeeding while at home, then start infant formula use when it's time to go back to work.

Still others struggle with the details of continuing to breastfeed after maternity leave is over – where to find a breast pump, the ability to afford a breast pump, how to work pumping into the workday, fear about not expressing enough breast milk, fear about the ability to continue producing enough breastmilk, finding a breastfeeding-friendly child care provider, as well as the challenge of working with her employer to have time and privacy to pump.

How do you help African-American mothers successfully return to the workplace while continuing to breastfeed?

Be Realistic

Have you ever put together a bookcase or an item from IKEA without the instructions? Did you happen to simply look at the picture and think, "Oh, I get it." Somehow the end product had leftover parts, and you scratched your head wondering, "How?" Did you use your hand to turn the screws, instead of the Alan wrench that was included? Thinking back, once you looked at the finished product, you didn't have realistic expectations. The same holds true when trying to convince African-American women that returning to work while breastfeeding is an attainable goal. Here are some tips to help you convince her:

1. Communicate to your client that if she has breastfed for one day, one month, three months, six months, one year, she has the resiliency to continue to breastfeed and to express her breastmilk upon return to the workplace.

2. Don't sell her dreams that it will be easy. Instead, help her make a realistic plan on how returning to work and continuing to breastfeed can be successful.

3. Impart this wisdom: Have a sense of humor. Expect the unexpected and laugh about it.

Help her Communicate with her Employer Before Going on Maternity Leave

It's critical to help your African-American client understand the importance of communicating with her employer about her decision to breastfeed. It's not important for her to get permission from her employer to breastfeed. That is not the point here. Due to returning to work being one of the major barriers to breastfeeding in the African-American community, it's important to communicate with the employer before hand to break this myth. By speaking with her employer in advance of maternity leave, she will feel empowered and more confident that things will work well upon return to work.

Things To Share With her Employer

Benefits to the employer:

- Fewer days off. A healthier child means fewer days off for mom.

- Happier employees equal a more productive workforce. When breastfeeding mothers are supported, they tend to be more focused at work.

- Good press. Companies that have good maternity policies and support breastfeeding cultivate a reputation of being mother-friendly.

- Sample letter to employer.

SAMPLE LETTER TO YOUR SUPERVISOR

TO: [Supervisor's name]

FROM: [Your name]

RE: Lactation support in the workplace

First, I want to thank you for your support during my [number] years with [company]. This is an exciting time for my family as we prepare for the birth of our child. I am eager to work with you to assure my productive return to work as soon as practicable after the birth of my baby.

Based on advice from my doctor and other health professionals, I have made the decision to breastfeed my baby. Just as I want to continue to give my best to the company, I also want to give the best I can to my baby. My doctor tells me that breastfeeding is important in preventing many illnesses and diseases for my baby and for me. Many employers across America now help make breastfeeding possible for working mothers. I hope we can find a mutually beneficial way to make breastfeeding possible when I am back at work.

If the company has an established lactation policy, I would like to know what it is so I can begin planning. If you want to understand better what is involved, you may want to start by looking at www. worksitesforwellness.org/foremployers.htm.

Thank you. Knowing that the company will help make it possible for me to continue breastfeeding will make me feel much better about leaving my baby home to come back to work. I look forward to discussing this with you.

[Your signature]

From: http://www.worksitesforwellness.org/letter-to-supervisor. html

Mom needs:

- Time to pump.
- Space to pump.
- Privacy and discretion.

- Consideration and mindfulness.

- Information that breastfeeding is vital to the health of her African-American baby: Breastfeeding is key to a healthy start in life.

- Education about breastpumps, storage, and how much milk she needs for her baby.

Help her Find a Breastfeeding-Friendly Childcare Provider

Have mom ask the childcare provider:

- Do you support breastfeeding?

- Did you breastfeed?

- Are there any other breastfed babies in your center?

- Breastmilk is different than infant formula. Are you willing to handle breastmilk differently?

- How will you feel about me breastfeeding my baby at the center?

- Will you handle my breastmilk per my instructions?

Guiding Principle: Provide adequate groundwork for effectively returning to work.

Chapter Eleven.
Outreach

As you know, outreach is the act of providing health information and services to communities that have poor health disparities. Outreach plans help to change these disparities by targeting communities and offering services in a strategic and culturally appropriate manner. For outreach to be successful, target groups must buy into the message that is offered, thus the messenger must be mindful and vigilant of cultural norms; barriers to healthcare and insurance; and social, economic, and institutional hindrances to change.

Outreach to the African-American Community

It's important to make outreach to the African-American community a regular practice. But how do you provide effective outreach to African-American women? You can design an outreach plan and/or evaluate an existing plan to consider what is going well and what needs improvement.

Have budget limitations? Often breastfeeding outreach is limited by budget, hospital regulations, or federal and state mandates. Don't let your budget stop you from reaching your goals. By planning ahead and being creative, you can effectively promote breastfeeding to African-American women.

Importance of Planning

Plan ahead. Review what has been done in the past in the area of outreach in general, then specifically target African-American women. Review what has worked and what has not been so successful.

Goals and Objectives of Your Hospital, Agency, or Organization

In developing goals and objectives, look at what works outside of your own organization. Research organizations and agencies, such as WIC, Health and Human Services, African American Breastfeeding Alliance, International Center for Traditional Child Rearing, Mocha Moms, Mocha Manual, and other resources you find on the Internet. Reach out to leaders in the African-American community who have been trailblazers in the area of breastfeeding outreach for advice and leadership.

Think Outside the Box

- Reach out to African-American churches for assistance and program support.

- Contact local chapters of Black sororities. They are always looking for programs to support in the community.

- Contact the free media. Send information about your services to the calendar section of free newspapers in your city.

- Hold your support groups or breastfeeding classes at libraries in Black communities or at local historical Black universities.

- Step outside of your organization or hospital and collaborate with a hospital with a high African-American birthrate. Offer to hold free breastfeeding classes.

Elements of the Plan

1. Goals

2. Target

3. Tune into Station WIFT: What's In It For Them?

4. Program

5. Outcome

6. Resources

Outreach Do's

- RESPECT = an open door.

- Have professional objectivity.

- Be flexible.

- Understand cultural factors that lead to non-responsiveness and how culture impacts decision-making.

- Practice nonjudgmental attitudes and behaviors.

- Recognize appropriate/inappropriate engagement.

Outreach Don'ts

- Patronize.

- Pretend while reaching out and being out in the community.

- Sell dreams.

- Argue with other lactation professionals about outreach plans or goals.

- Burnout. Take time for yourself and recognize when you are patronizing, pretending, selling dreams, or arguing.

Evaluate all activities and tweak your plan until you get it right. Remember: Right is what works for the women you serve.

Guiding Principle: Implement outreach to the African-American community as a regular practice.

Chapter Twelve.
Survey Results

I conducted a short survey of a broad spectrum of African-American lactation professionals. Fifteen responded. They are IBCLCs, peer counselors, CLCs, pediatricians, neonatologists, RNs, and public health professionals. These professionals:

- Are located in over ten different states, in every region of the country.

- Work in hospitals, birth centers, doctor's offices, WIC agencies, government and non-profit programs, and healthcare environments.

- Have over 50 years combined experience managing lactation problems and promoting breastfeeding in the African-American community.

Below is an overview of the most important questions and answers that are relevant to this book. Some comments may surprise you. I assure you, however, these insights will help you, in a quick and tactical way, understand your African-American clients, reach Black women, and manage your clients more effectively.

The Diversity of African-American Women Served

Please describe in detail the cultural, social, economic, and political demographics of the women you've provided lactation consulting to over the years.

- I provide counseling and breastfeeding support to a variety of families within the African-American community. I've counseled teen moms, married women and their husbands, and single mothers. Also, my families' income varies from low-income to higher middle-class.

- For the past three years, I have worked primarily with African-American mothers who are WIC-eligible and Medicaid-eligible in a hospital setting and offer early post-partum breastfeeding assistance. Many are from different cultures and social economic groups.

- I work with urban "inner-city" African-Americans, WIC-based populations across the income eligibility spectrum; immigrant African, Central/South-American, Spanish speaking, Caribbean; middle to upper income, urban and suburban African-American and Caucasian; European, Asian; public health, hospital based and private care - generally across a wide socio-economic, cultural, and political range.

- I work with women of African descent from various social-economic backgrounds. Yet, they tend to be of a similar socio-cultural background. Many women that I service happen to qualify for WIC.

- Our area is mostly African-American and Hispanic. Low socioeconomic area, education levels are low, and some women are first generation breast feeders. So support is also low.

- Teens-Single Parent Homes-Christian-Democrats-Republicans-Working mothers-Unemployed-TANF-Lesbians

- I have provided lactation consulting to women of every cultural, social, economic, and political demographic. African-American women, Latinos, Indian, Caucasian, economically and socially disadvantaged, as well as upper class women, democrats, republicans, and independents.

- I do not provide lactation consulting. Soul Food for Your Baby provides support to African-American/Black women at all socioeconomic levels, but primarily focuses on support to low-income women.

- I work at a hospital near downtown Detroit. We deliver a lot of high-risk mothers-approximately 6,000 deliveries/year. We have a significant African-American population, of which a good deal have Medicaid/WIC.

- I work with low-income African-American women from WIC.

- I have worked with mothers in the WIC population for over 17 years, so they have been as young as 12 years old to 45 years old. They have been very poor, with no resources to working mothers and fathers.

- Primarily low income, Medicaid-enrolled African-American women. I also provide consultation to professional colleagues and friends free of charge.

- African-American and the general population of women in low- to moderate-income brackets, with first to many pregnancies.

Addressing Cultural, Social, and Economic Issues

Culture plays an important role in influencing African-American women to breastfeed. The following advice is tried and true.

What advice do you offer your clients about how to address cultural issues (history of breastfeeding, family practices, belief about infant formula, etc.?)

- Seek out women with a similar cultural background who can share their experiences with overcoming barriers.

- Discuss the disparities in health and the mortality rate for Blacks compared to other races. Encourage women to be aware of their health.

- I discuss the history of breastfeeding in U.S. and why it is not prevalent in the Black culture, why formula is available and easy to access vs. breastfeeding support. I provide counseling geared toward understanding and resolving internal or cultural barriers, including family members in breastfeeding classes and management sessions.

- We share the U.S. history of breastfeeding for African-Americans. The intent is to make mothers aware of their history and to let them know that we come from a tradition of breastfeeding women that has been tangled up in this booby trap throughout history in the U.S.

- I address cultural myths that are based on lies, cultural hurts, and personal biases. I find educating grandparents helps a lot in providing support for the breastfeeding family, as they can be the best advocates.

- Don't be discouraged by anyone else's opinion. You do what you feel is best for your baby. No one is perfect and it's okay to make a mistake or to choose something different.

- Understand origination of non-breastfeeding among African-Americans, history of breastfeeding, and discrediting of the myths.

- Breastfeeding is empowering because moms know they are providing the best nourishment for their babies. This is encouraging when confronted with stares or negative comments. Women are continuing a natural legacy long performed by their African ancestors.

- You CAN be the first in your family to breastfeed.

- You are not alone.

- Bottles are not easier.

- In the beginning – no formula, no bottles. It's species specific. Birth control and spacing children in other cultures. Health issues for the African-Americans population.

Social Issues and Advice From the Field

Breastfeeding is one of those parenting areas where everyone, at least in the U.S., wants to feel normal. No one wants to be seen breastfeeding in public or breastfeeding a toddler. In the African-American community, normalizing breastfeeding as much as possible is key to breastfeeding promotion and success.

What advice do you offer your clients about how to address social issues (lack of family support, lack of role models, etc.)?

- Seek out breastfeeding mothers in the community.

- Attend groups where other women who breastfeed are attending. Create a group for women of color to meet and share concerns.

- Refer to support groups; provide print material/videos targeting other family members/friends; refer to providers/support persons from similar background.

- Commune with a group of women who you can relate to, typically women of similar socio-cultural backgrounds.

- Education, education, and education! You have to understand why you're doing what you're doing and what the pay off is to you, your baby, and your family.

- Build a support team before the baby comes/don't be ashamed to allow people to assist you. You can choose whoever you want to be your supporter.

- More faith-based community support.

- Educating family members, specifically grandparents and fathers.

- Include dads, grandmothers, friends, and/or others in the breastfeeding process and with baby care, childcare, and housework. Join WIC, a breastfeeding support group, or a mom's group.

- Try to find someone that will support you in breastfeeding - a friend, family member, church member – and talk with them.

- Talk to your family about breastmilk and your decision on nursing your baby.

- As a Lactation Professional, you have to constantly check up on the mom, especially in the first two weeks, share the stories and experiences you have had working with mothers, cheer her on, and address her concerns. Let her know that she will change the thinking of someone else in her circle through her experience and provide her with lots of encouragement and accolades.

- I tend to provide examples of non-nutritive means of providing support that family members can offer.

- The more support you have the better, bring to class support system, get to know other African-American women at group meetings and find out how they were successful.

Helping Your Clients Understand Economic Barriers

What advice do you offer your clients about how to address economic barriers, such as returning to work, childcare, etc.?

- Identify resources.

- Where you can obtain a pump if returning to work or school.

- Provide resources – information, references to pumps, communication with employers, and assistance with establishing pumping/feeding schedules. Provide *pro bono* services when necessary.

- We offer mothers free hand pumps and make electric pumps available at a low price. We also write letters on behalf of mothers to their employers regarding breastfeeding or offer suggestions about how to address the issue with their employers. Peers share their ideas and experiences with economic barriers to other moms.

- Again, education and available support to the breastfeeding family. I try to be very diligent in educating my families about laws and best practices surrounding their right to breastfeeding. I work with my families to find suppliers in their area so their experience with breastfeeding upon returning to work is as free from stress as possible. Having my own list of resources has been very helpful in referring my families to retailers and others in this field.

- Seek out funding for agency staffing, supplies, and training to provide adequate support to my clients and offer free resources within the community.

- Providing pumps and showing the actual money saved.

- It is important to discuss pumping at work during the prenatal period because preparation is important for return-to-work success. Many employers try to accommodate the needs of breastfeeding employees to some degree. Pumps are available to moms if they are on WIC.

- Provide education on all the different types of breastpumps. Let her know that you get what you pay for when buying a cheap pump, which usually equals poor quality. Provide education on hand expression.

- Talking to your employer about the benefits for them, as well as for yourself before leaving on maternity leave. Discuss with the employer – access to a place for pumping, milk storage, and time to pump.

- I encourage women to approach their employers early to discuss their needs upon returning to work, explore options for obtaining pumps through WIC or Medicaid, and offer assistance with letters to insurers and employers.

- Establish milk first if possible before returning to work or school. Find a daycare that supports breastfeeding.

- Discuss with employer the possibility of creating a Breastfeeding-Friendly workplace. WIC provides a pump to those on WIC without insurance that will pay for a pump. Anticipatory guidance to returning to work or school.

- Communication – Perhaps the Most Important Tip of All!

Guiding Principle: Recognize trusted methods of lactation counseling.

Conclusion

Why did you read this book? Why did you make it to the conclusion? Or, why did you skip past all the details in the previous chapters to make it to the end, the bottom line?

Chances are you are a dedicated and enthusiastic lactation professional. You are skilled at what you do – providing excellent breastfeeding management, education, and support to the women in your practice or agency.

It's likely that for the past several years your clients have been changing – they're more racially and economically diverse. With more African-American clients and the knowledge that breastfeeding promotion, education, and management are not a one-size fits all approach, it's important to use all the resources available.

Why is breastfeeding a health imperative for African-Americans? Since we have some of the highest rates of, and death due to, the following illnesses, breastfeeding is vital to:

- Improve health for African-American babies.

- Reduce SIDS, asthma, and obesity.

- Reduce the infant mortality rate. African Americans have 2.4 times the infant mortality rate as non-Hispanic whites.

- Reduce prematurity – 18.1% of African-American babies are born premature.

- Create a healthy lifestyle for African-American mothers.

- Decrease rates of cancer.

- Decrease obesity.

- Increase self-empowerment.

For the past 20 years, researchers, government agencies, and breastfeeding advocates have been considering the African-American breastfeeding mixed-conundrum:

- Why do breastfeeding rates among African-American women fall far behind other races?

- What makes overcoming breastfeeding barriers more difficult for

Black women?

- Why are breastfeeding promotion programs more challenging in the African-American community?

- How can lactation professionals provide more culturally competent care to African-American mothers?

While breastfeeding rates have been slow to increase, not quite meeting Healthy People 2010 and other government set goals, the good news is that more Black women are breastfeeding and more organizations exist to support breastfeeding in African-American communities. There are more African-American IBCLC's today than ever before.

Unfortunately, this is not enough. The need for lactation professionals to have the proper tools to assist Black mothers with breastfeeding management, provide education, and promote breastfeeding is still a major concern and priority. The major issues that negatively impact a Black woman's decision to breastfeed include:

- History

- Shift in cultural belief in importance and spiritual nature of breastfeeding

- Demise of breastfeeding tradition

- Change in dynamics of Black family

- Birth practices

- Belief in breastfeeding myths

- High level of infant formula marketing in Black neighborhoods

As a lactation consultant, you can read many books and go to hundreds of lectures on Black women and breastfeeding, but to be effective in reaching Black women is relatively simple:

- Have an open mind.

- Decide to make a difference.

- Make mom's end goal, THE goal.

- Remember – your end result is irrelevant.

- Seek answers from the Black mothers you serve.

- Work with other Black IBCLCs and peer counselors – they will teach you much from the field.

- Know that RESPECT equals an open door.

- Always maintain professional objectivity.

- Understand cultural factors.

- Practice nonjudgmental attitudes and behaviors.

- Recognize appropriate/inappropriate engagement.

- Never ever use colloquialisms that you don't use in your regular everyday speech.

Take one client at a time, one mom at a time, and realize that you can make a difference in the health and well-being of your African-American mothers and babies.

References

AAP Section on Breastfeeding. (2012). Breastfeeding and the use of human milk. *Pediatrics, 129*(3), e827-e841.

American Cancer Society. (2012). *Breast cancer overview.* Retrieved from: http://www.cancer.org/cancer/breastcancer/overviewguide/breast-cancer-overview-what-causes

Bentley, M.E., Caulfield, L.E, Gross, S.M., Bronner, Y., Jensen, J., Kessler, L.A., & Paige, D.M. (1999). Sources of influence on intention to breastfeed among African-American women at entry to WIC. *J Hum Lact, 15*(1), 27-34.

Bureau of Labor and Statistics. (2012). *Labor force characteristics by race and ethnicity.* Report 1036. Retrieved from: http://www.bls.gov/cps/cpsrace2011.pdf.

CDC. (2012). *Provisional breastfeeding rates by socio-demographic factors, among children born in 2007 (percent +/- half 95% confidence interval).* Retrieved from: http://www.cdc.gov/breastfeeding/data/NIS_data/2007/socio-demographic_any.htm

Cricco-Lizza, R. (2006). Black non-Hispanic mothers' perceptions about the promotion of infant-feeding methods by nurses and physicians. *J Obstet Gynecol Neonatal Nurs, 35*(2), 173-80.

DHHS (U.S. Department of Health & Human Services). (2012a). *Childhood obesity.* Retrieved from: http://aspe.hhs.gov/health/reports/child_obesity/

DHHS. (2012b). Minority women's health. *Breast cancer.* Retrieved from: http://www.womenshealth.gov/minority-health/african-americans/breast-cancer.cfm.

Giugliani, E.R.J., Bronner, Y., Caiaffa, W.T., Vogelhut, J., Witter, F.R., & Perman, J.A. (1994). Are fathers prepared to encourage their partners to breastfeed? *Acta Paediatrica 83,* 1127-31.

MacDorman, M.F., & Mathews, T.J. (2008). *Recent trends in infant mortality in the United States. NCHS data brief, no 9.* Hyattsville, MD: National Center for Health Statistics.

Morrison, T. (2006). *Beloved.* New York: Everyman's Library.

National Heart Lung and Blood Institute. (2012). *Reducing asthma disparities.* Retrieved from: http://www.nhlbi.nih.gov/health/prof/lung/asthma/naci/discover/disparities.htm.

Thompson, A.L., & Bentley, M.E. (2012). The critical period of infant feeding for the development of early disparities in obesity. *Soc Sci Med.* pii: S0277-9536(12)00814-3. doi: 10.1016/j.socscimed.2012.12.007.

Wolfberg, A.J., Michels, K.B., Shields, W., O'Campo, P., Bronner, Y., & Bienstock, J. (2004). Dads as breastfeeding advocates: results from a randomized controlled trial of an educational intervention. *Am J Obstet Gynecol, 191*(3), 708-12.

Bibliography

Barber, K. (2005). *The black woman's guide to breastfeeding: The definitive guide to nursing for African American mothers*. Naperville, IL: Sourcebooks.

Follett, R. (2003). Heat, sex and sugar: Pregnancy and childbearing in the slave quarters. *Journal of Family History, 28*(4), 510-539.

Preston, S.H., & Haines, M. (1991). *Fatal years: Child mortality in late nineteenth century America*. Princeton University Press, pp. 26-29.

Thomas, V.G. (2004). The psychology of black women: Studying women's lives in context. *Journal of Black Psychology, 30*(3), 286-306.

Resources

Websites

Black Women Do Breastfeed

http://blackwomendobreastfeed.wordpress.com/

Blacktating Breastfeeding News and Views from a Mom of Color

www.blacktating.com

Mocha Manual.com Motherhood in Color

http://mochamanual.com

Black Mothers' Breastfeeding Association

http://blackmothersbreastfeeding.org/

Handouts / Publications

Your Guide to Breastfeeding for African American Women

http://www.womenshealth.gov/publications/our-publications/
breastfeeding-guide/BreastfeedingGuide-AfricanAmerican-English.
pdf

Articles

Beyonce breastfeeding controversy: What does it mean to black moms?

http://thegrio.com/2012/03/07/beyonce-breastfeeding-controversy-
what-does-it-mean-to-black-moms/#s:beyonce_baby_breastfeeding_
4x3-jpg

About the Author

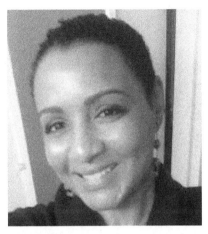

While successfully nursing her son in the late 1990's, Kathi Barber became intrigued with breastfeeding. She began to read about breastfeeding and came across the startling statistics about breastfeeding in the Black community. Kathi took training courses with La Leche League and other groups, which led her to become immersed in the breastfeeding sub-culture. This was not sufficient for her, however, because the breastfeeding sub-culture was largely white. Kathi was passionately compelled to help women in her own African-American community. In January of 2000, she established the African American Breastfeeding Alliance (AABA), the first non-profit organization whose sole mission was to support breastfeeding in the Black community, and educate Black families and their support people (i.e., doctors, LC's, WIC staff, nurses, etc.) about the importance of breastfeeding in this population.

As Founder and Executive Director of AABA, Kathi has spoken nationally to hundreds of professionals, organizations, agencies and mothers on breastfeeding and African-American women. She is regularly approached by the media when a new statistic or research study is released and Black women and breastfeeding are involved. In the mid-2000's, former Surgeon General Dr. David Satcher commended her efforts at an international breastfeeding conference of over a thousand attendees. In early 2003, her work was featured in a two-page article in the *Washington Post*. Years of passionate effort on the behalf of the women in her community led her to write the first book on breastfeeding and Black women – *The Black Woman's Guide to Breastfeeding: The Definitive Guide to Nursing for African American Mothers*, published by Sourcebooks in 2005.

CPSIA information can be obtained
at www.ICGtesting.com
Printed in the USA
LVHW022136020120
642358LV00010B/165